Back Pain Relief Exercises And Stretches

For

Seniors

Best Exercises for Chronic Lower Back Pain, Improved Mobility, Joint Health, Balance, Pain Relief, and Injury Prevention

Owen Brown

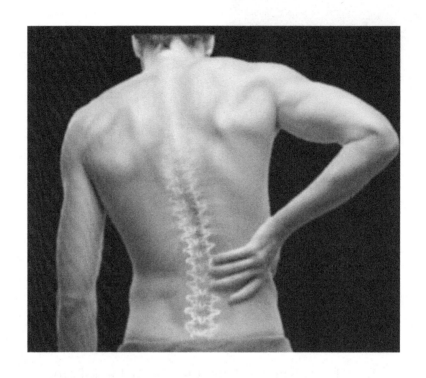

Table of Contents

Introduction

Lower back protection and regular exercise are essential for seniors to feel safe and secure when they walk, sit or stand at home.

For elderly people, a spinal injury can have life-altering implications because every movement the body makes starts with the spine.

The spine and lower back are held stable by a slew of small muscles that collaborate to produce the subtle movements necessary for balance. Elderly people who want to maintain their independence should do back strengthening exercises.

Some back strengthening workouts are not suitable for seniors. To keep the lower back in place while other muscles around it are stretched, back workouts should always include a stabilizing component.

For instance, a good lower back workout stretches the muscles behind the leg but keeps the lower back stable and engaged. It is in this way that leg movement strengthens the lower back and spinal muscles learn to contract and create stability.

If these exercises cause any discomfort, the patient should stop and consult with a medical professional.

Part 1

How Often Should Seniors Perform Back Strengthening Exercises?

It is recommended that back strengthening exercises be performed at least three times per week to improve an elderly person's balance and mobility, but more frequently is preferable. However, if your back feels tired or sore after a workout, take a break between sessions to avoid aggravating it.

To Keep Their Backs Healthy, What Exercises Should Seniors Avoid?

The use of heavyweights and back stretches involving hyperextension are generally not recommended for seniors. Seniors who want to strengthen their backs should carry out regular, gentle workouts that target the core and keep the back's smaller muscles engaged. Stretching workouts that involve bouncing should also be avoided.

People over the age of 65 should avoid the following exercises:

1. Weight training (squats with dumbbells, bench press, leg press, etc.)
2. Running for long distances
3. Abdominal crunches and sit-ups
4. Upright rowing
5. High-intensity interval training
6. Rock climbing

What Causes Low Back Pain?

Low back pain is the fifth most common reason for a doctor's visit in the United States.

It is estimated that over 85% of these visits are for low back pain that cannot be traced to a specific disease or abnormality in the spine.

There are several possible causes of nonspecific back pain, including but not limited to:

Muscle Spasms

Muscle Strains

Nerve Injuries

Degenerative Changes

Some specific and more serious causes of back pain include:

Compression Fractures

Spinal Stenosis

Disc Herniation

Cancer

Infection

Spondylolisthesis

Neurological Disorders

Part 2

Start Strong

Our bodies are at their most efficient when all of our muscles work together.

Back pain or injury can occur if you have weak muscles in your core and pelvis.

Having low back pain can make it difficult to go about your daily routine. Strengthening exercises are beneficial in the treatment of lower back pain.

The best way to avoid low back pain is to lead a healthy lifestyle. When it comes to preventing low back pain as you get older, it's important to keep your weight down, build strength, and avoid risky activities.

The muscles that support your spine can be strengthened with these simple exercises.

Strengthening your muscles can help alleviate pain and discomfort.

According to the American Chiropractic Association, back pain is the second most common reason people visit their doctor.

Even if you don't have arthritis or other debilitating health conditions, you may still experience back pain. There is no evidence that back pain is caused by an infection, fracture, or any other serious condition, as the American Chiropractic Association (ACA) states. Inner-body issues like kidney stones or blood clots rarely cause back pain.

In many cases, this means that treating or preventing back pain at home is an option. Even more importantly, as we age, maintaining strong postural muscles and a flexible spine, as well as moving in ways that support our backs, are two of the best ways to keep back pain at bay. Stretching is an easy way to accomplish all of this. Before attempting these stretches, make an appointment with your doctor or physical therapist, especially if you are experiencing back pain.

What Do I Need

A sturdy chair, like a dining room chair, should be used for all of the exercises below, preferably not an armchair. Sitting on a more rigid surface will make it easier to maintain good posture. Nothing else is needed. To start, you want to make sure you have your feet firmly on the ground, your knees bent at a 90-degree angle, and you are sitting square in the seat, not perched on the edge of it.

Stretches To Relief Back Pain
Neck And Chest Stretch

In the days before screens became so ubiquitous, people used to regularly tuck their chins in to read, eat (when they look at their plates), drive, and do a variety of other activities that required them to tuck their chins in. There is a link between neck pain and other parts of the spine and back, especially the upper and middle spine. This exercise helps to loosen up the chest, which can become constrictive due to poor posture and needs to be reopened.

This stretches your scapulae and trapezius muscles in your neck, as well as your pectorals and erector spinae, and gently works your oblique muscles.

Steps

- Sit with your feet flat on the floor and your back straight to get started. As you breathe in and out, place your hands at the base of your skull with your fingers intertwined and thumbs running down your neck. (The "relaxing, laid back" pose, with your head resting in your hands, is a classic example.)

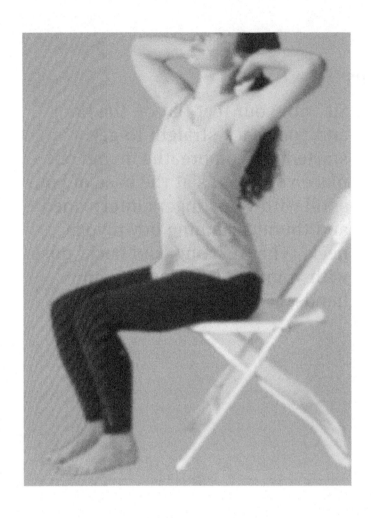

- Raise your chin to your chest and
  look up at the ceiling as you slowly
  lower your head into your palms.

- Take a deep breath in. Relax your
  left elbow toward the floor and your

right elbow toward the ceiling as you exhale. Your neck will benefit from a well-supported stretch. It's fine if your elbows only move an inch or two in this movement, as long as it's an easy one. A good stretch, not a painful one, is what you're looking for.

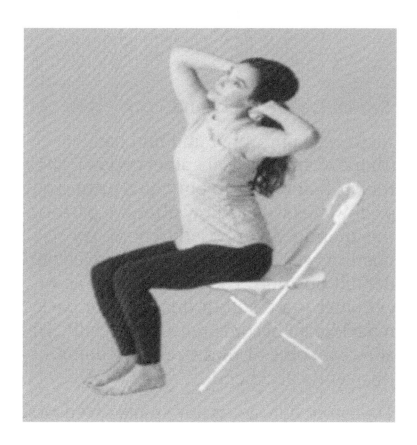

- Relax your spine and take 2 deep breaths.

- Repeat on the other side, with the right elbow pointing down and the left elbow pointing up. Do this three times on each side, then switch sides.

Seated Gentle Backbend

As we age, our upper and mid-back (thoracic and cervical spine) curve forward more due to our chins jutting out or down, as well as how often we perform this motion. As opposed to our "lazy" posture, we can adopt this posture as our default position. The hunch we get as we get older is a result of this, and our back muscles can become tense as a result. To alleviate some of that stress, try doing this gentle backbend.

This stretch targets your spinal extensors, anterior neck muscles, and pectoral muscles.

Steps:

- Assume a seated position, place your hands on your lower back with your fingers facing down and your thumbs wrapped around your hips toward your front body.

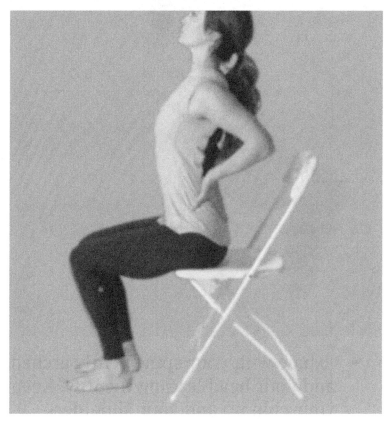

- You can do this by firmly pressing your hands into your hips/lower back and inhaling.

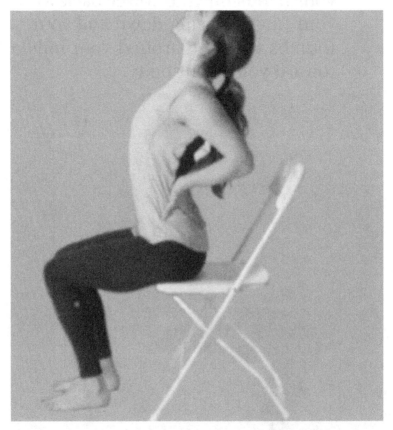

- Exhale with your spine gently arched and your head leading the way. Keep your chin up and your shoulders back. The cervical spine is where you'll want to take the lead, so gently tilting your chin up and facing the ceiling is a good place to start. The upper and mid-spine should be involved in the backbend, not just the lower back.

- Hold the pose for five full, deep breaths.

- Repeat 3 - 6 times, returning slowly and carefully to the initial position.

Reach Back

In addition to stretching your shoulders and chest, this stretch improves your range of motion. Sitting or standing with our shoulders slumped can make us feel as if we're relaxing into a slouch. As a result, our chests become inflamed from the effort required to draw those muscles inward. By avoiding the use of those muscles, it can also lead to discomfort in the upper and mid-back.

The following exercise stretches the chest, strengthens the back, and increases the range of motion in the shoulders.

This stretch is particularly beneficial for your anterior deltoids, as well as your pectorals. Muscles worked:

Steps:

- Straighten your spine and keep your feet firmly planted on the ground. Take a deep breath in, and as you exhale, clasp your hands together behind your back. Make sure to grab the opposite wrists or elbows instead of intertwining your hands if you are unable to.

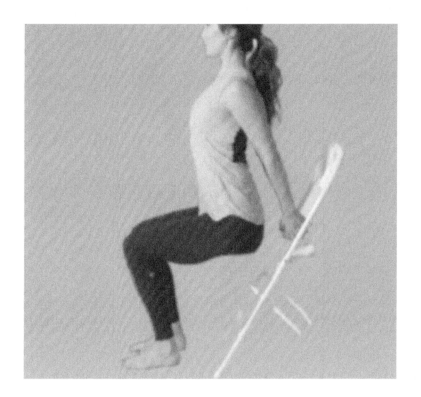

- Take a deep breath again and notice how your spine lengthens as you sit up straighter. Move your shoulder blades downward as you raise and lower your shoulders.

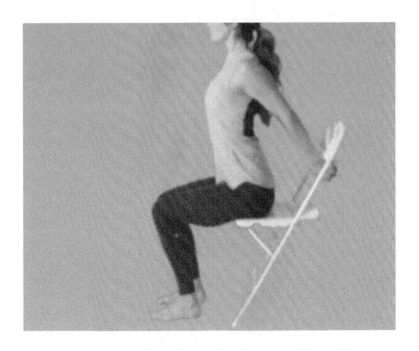

- If your hands are clasped, gently straighten your arms. (If your hands aren't clasped, gently pull them apart.) Your upper back will be opened up as a result of this.

- Release your grip after taking a couple of deep breaths, and then go back to neutral.

- Repeat this three times.

Take it to the next level

To ensure that nothing is being strained, you should feel comfortable increasing the stretch to include the entire spine. In addition to relieving your lower back pain, it can also improve your spinal mobility.

Steps:

- To begin, begin by clasping your hands behind your back or gripping the opposite wrist or elbow of the person next to you.

- Feel your ribs rise and your spine lengthen as you inhale. Gently bend forward at the waist as if you were bringing your ribs to your thighs while maintaining that spine-tingling sensation.

- Only go so far as you're comfortable with. Even if you can get all the way down to your thighs, don't rest your weight on them. Keep your postural muscles engaged as you stretch your chest, shoulders, and back.

Seated Cat-Cow

Many people experience pain in the lower back. Osteoarthritis and spinal degeneration are becoming more common as we get older. When we have bad posture, we may also stand with a "flat pelvis," which can lead to a lot of lower back pain. Cat-Cow is a great exercise for stretching and strengthening lower back muscles, as well as a good way to keep the spine in good shape.

There are a lot of muscles involved in this exercise, including erector spinae; serratus anterior; the iliac bone; and the muscles of the abdominals (rectus abdominis).

Steps:

- To begin, stand with your feet flat on the floor and your knees bent at a 90-degree angle. Place your hands on your knees, palms facing in and heels on the outside of your legs.

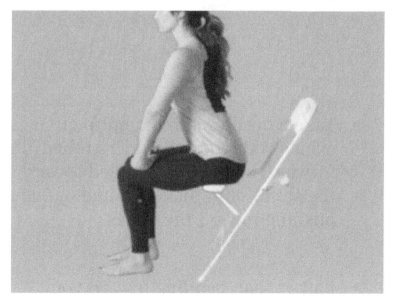

- Exhale while pressing your hands into your sides and arching your back from the base of your neck to your head. Face the sky and feel as if you're pressing your butt out in the back of your chair.

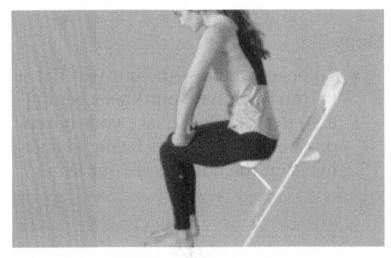

- Take a deep breath in and then exhale with your shoulders rolled forward, belly button pulled toward the spine, chin tucked in and hands pushing toward the knees.

- Rather than bending toward your knees on your next exhalation, reverse the motion by pulling the chest through the arms and arching the spine again.

- Take a few breaths and repeat this 3 - 6 times.

Gentle twist

While twisting your spine lightly has numerous health benefits, it is also one of the most effective stretches for relieving lower back pain. In addition, twisting your spine a few times a day can help prevent lower back pain in the future.

There are several muscles in your neck and upper back that are worked during this stretch as well (such as sternocleidomastoid and splenius capitis).

Steps:

- Begin with your knees bent at a 90-degree angle and your feet flat on the floor. Edge the seat forward just a tad bit. A little more room behind you is nice, but you don't want to feel like the chair is tipping forward or unstable.

- As you take a deep breath in, sit up straight, lengthening your spine, and raise your arms overhead.

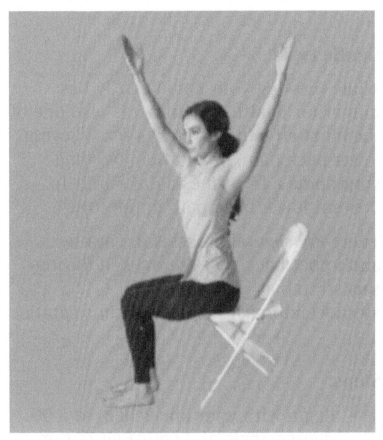

- Exhale and turn slightly to the right, placing your left hand on the outside of your right knee and your right hand wherever is most comfortable. Do not use that hand to "crank" your twist any further by placing it on the seat or back of the chair. Using your arm strength to twist yourself more forcefully can lead to injury and an uneven amount of twisting in different parts of your spine.

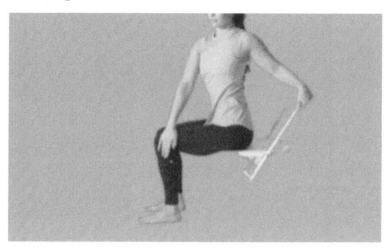

- Hold the twist and lift your torso higher as you inhale. Twist a little deeper as you exhale.

- Hold the twist for 3 to 5 breaths before releasing it and repeating the exercise on the other side. Stretch on each side at least twice, then switch sides and do the same thing the other way around.

Part 3

Back Strengthening Exercises for Seniors

Bent Knee Raise

The bent knee raise is a good workout for seniors who are just starting. A minimal amount of time and effort is required to accomplish this simple but effective workout. Increasing the strength in your abs and lower back is one of the main benefits of this exercise. It can help you move more fluidly and alleviate pain associated with lumbar instability if you do it regularly.

Steps:

- After lying on your back with your knees bent and palms facing each other, perform the supine bent knee raise. If necessary, you can prop your head up on a pillow. A small pillow or blanket can be placed under the arch of your lower back to keep your tummy pressed forward and your core muscles engaged.

- Slowly raise one knee toward your chest. Don't go any further than you're comfortable with.

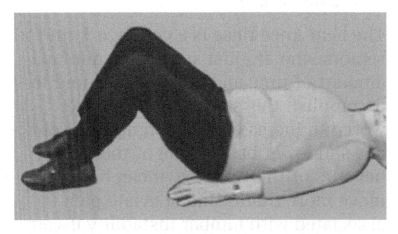

- Raise the other knee toward your chest and bring it into contact with the other knee.

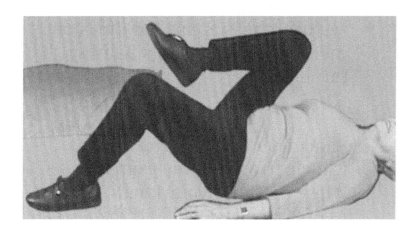

- Raise both of your legs to your chest for five seconds, then bring them back to their starting positions.

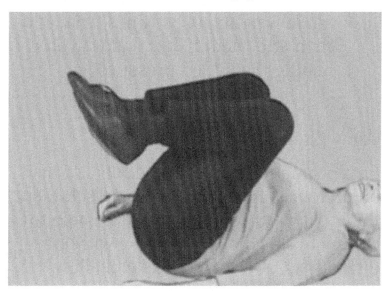

- Perform the exercise ten times on each leg, switching legs halfway through.

- Remember to take deep breaths while performing the exercise. When you raise your knees, it's best to breathe deeply in and then exhale as you bring them back to the ground. Wearing ankle weights that weigh 1 or 2 pounds per pair of feet can make this exercise more difficult. Do this workout without ankle weights a few times first, and then add them if you're sure you can handle the added pressure.

Cat & Camel

Cat & camel stretch for beginners focus on abdominal and hip flexor muscles. For the most part, seniors should be able to complete this simple exercise without difficulty. Cat & camel aids will allow elderly people to keep or regain their ability to turn and maneuver without fear of falling over. It's even better to do this exercise every day rather than three to five times a week.

A workout mat or other soft surface can be used in place of the ground if you prefer to perform this exercise on your bed rather than the ground. Hands shoulder-width apart, fingers facing forward, with knees slightly apart is the ideal position. At this point, your back should be straight.

Steps:

- As you arch back and lift the top of your head, keep your abdominal muscles engaged and your eyes focused upward (if possible). If any part of your body causes you pain or discomfort, stop and take a breather.

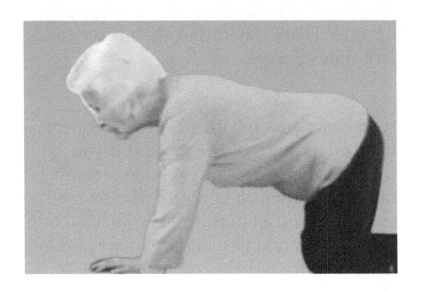

- Next, lower your head to the ground (or, even better, to your belly button and legs!) and bend your back so that it curves upwards. Always be mindful of your physical sensations and keep your abdominal muscles active.

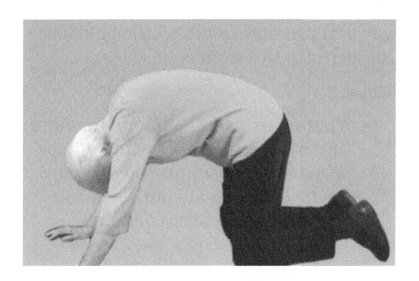

- Repeat this moves ten times. Breathe in while arching your back and out while bending it backward.

Bridging

Bridging is an easy workout that targets both the abs and the lower back while also targeting the core. Also, you'll be able to flex your hip flexors and increase your range of motion. To get the most out of this exercise, you'll need to do it 3 to 5 times a week. Anyone regardless of age or physical condition, with a little guidance, can perform this exercise.

Steps:

- Your feet should be flat on the floor and bent at the knees with the hips in a neutral position. You should keep your arms at your sides and not cross them over your chest.

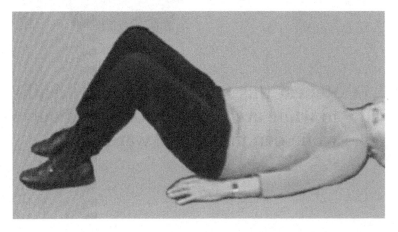

- Lift your bottom gradually until it is no longer touching the floor.

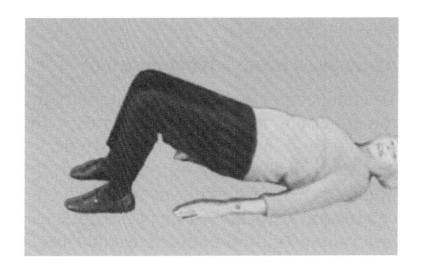

- Slowly lower yourself back to the mat by contracting your buttocks.

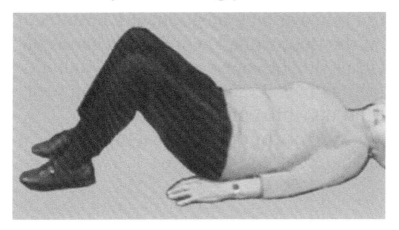

- To improve your strength to walk & stand, this workout can help you improve your balance.

Arm Raises (from a lying position)

To enhance posture as well as mobility in the upper and middle back, arm raises are a simple and highly effective way to do so. It is critical to have well-developed upper back and shoulder muscles, which can be quickly achieved by performing arm raises. To do this exercise, you can either lay down or sit down.

Steps:

Get into a supine position with both feet on the floor while keeping your hands on either side of your body with the palms facing down. You may want to prop your head up with a pillow. As an added measure of comfort, place a pillow or duvet under your lower back.

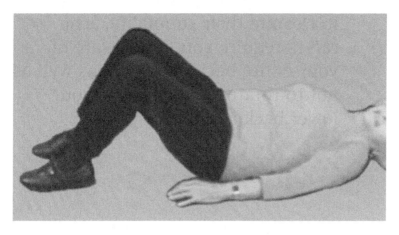

- Lie on your back and extend one arm straight out in front of you, with the hand straight out in front of your face. Bring it down gradually once more.

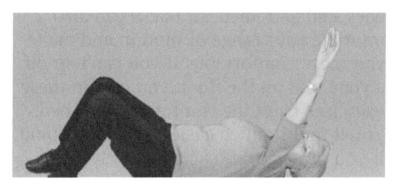

- Using the other arm, carry out the same exercise as you did before. For each arm, you will perform this exercise ten times.
- Inhale deeply as you raise your arm in a salute. Breathe out as you lower

it. Despite their simplicity, arm raises require you to be aware of your entire back and body, as well as not to rotate, turn or strain your lower back at all.

Sit-Backs

This exercise may be helpful for those of you who have trouble sitting down as well as standing up, or even getting out of bed. In addition to strengthening your back and abdomen, sit-backs can also improve your range of motion and make you more comfortable. If you can't sit on a yoga mat on the floor, you can do these exercises from the comfort of your bed. You'll find it much easier to sit and stand if you practice sit-backs regularly.

Steps:

- As you sit on the floor or in a bed, sit up straight & your knees bent. Cross your arms over your chest with your palms facing up and shoulders back. Be careful not to

overextend your knees, and
maintain a forward gaze at all times.

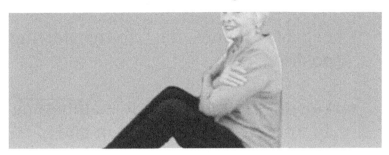

- Gradually lean back, making sure to
  lift with your core muscles.

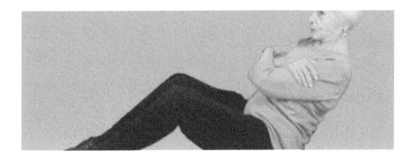

- Only walk as far as you feel safe,
  and don't push yourself to go any
  further than that for now. Make an
  effort to keep your back straight at
  all times.

- Repeat 10 times, back to the starting position.

- You should inhale while maintaining an upright seating position and exhale while leaning back when performing this movement. As you return to the seated position, take a deep breath in.

Standing Reverse Leg Lifts

It is a moderate-intensity exercise that focuses on the glutes, lower back, and lower abdominal muscles while standing on your toes In the long run, leg and lower body mobility will benefit from back exercises that incorporate the legs. As simple as it may seem, a standing reverse leg lift requires a strong and stable base. So don't give up on your reverse leg lift just yet!

Steps:

- With your legs hip-width apart, place your hands gently on a chair or countertop in front of you and begin to stand up straight and lean in. Throughout the exercise, make sure your shoulders are back and your chin is up.

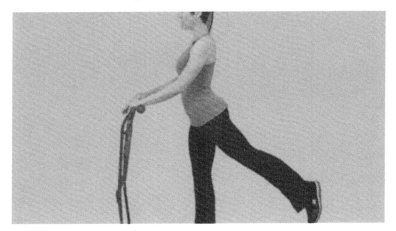

- Straighten one of your legs behind you. It's okay if you can only lift your leg a few centimeters off the floor the first time. Do what makes you feel most at ease.
- Hold this position for five full counts before gradually lowering your foot to the ground and

returning your leg to its starting position. Rep on the opposite side.

- On each leg, perform this exercise five times. Keep in mind that your abdominal muscles should be used for the majority of the lifting.

Warrior 2 Yoga Pose

A large number of senior citizens claim that yoga is extremely potent in reducing pain as well as improving their overall mobility and posture. This yoga pose is more challenging than other back-building exercises because it requires you to stand and work other muscles at the same time. If necessary, you can prop yourself up on a chair. Straight back and strong abdominal muscles are necessary for Warrior 2 yoga pose.

Steps:

- Begin by pointing your toes forward and spreading your feet wide (about two shoulder widths). Make sure your shoulders are back and your head is up at this point. Your arms should be resting at your sides, too.

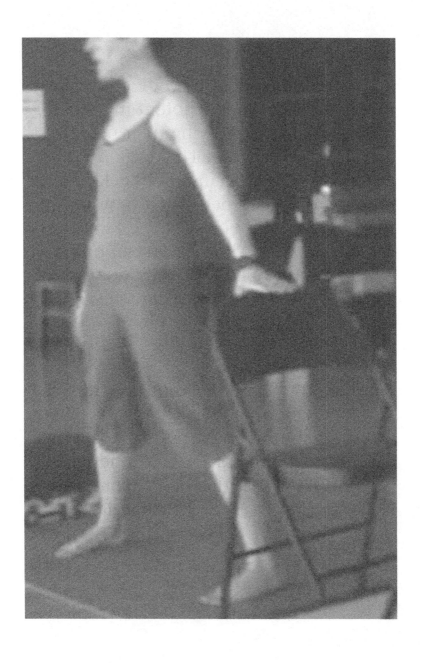

- Make a right turn with your right foot, pointing straight ahead with your toes. Raise your arms shoulder-height towards you.

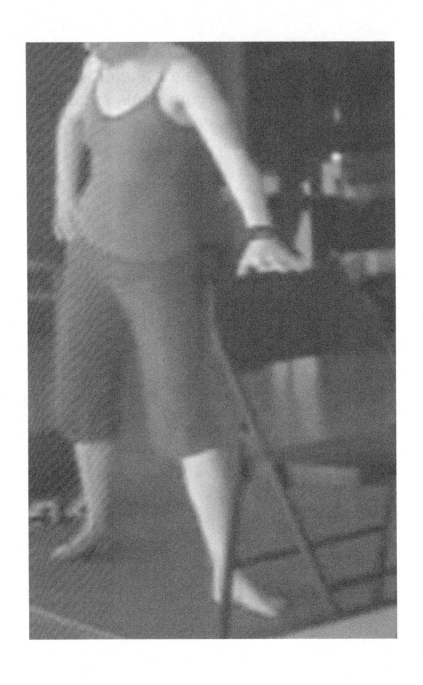

- Knees slightly bent (your left leg will stay straight). You should only bend your leg as far as is comfortable for you, and your knee should not extend past the big toe on your right foot at any point during the process.

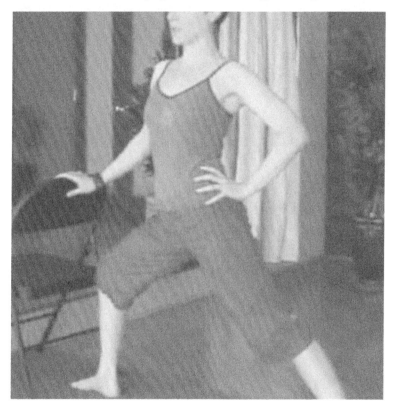

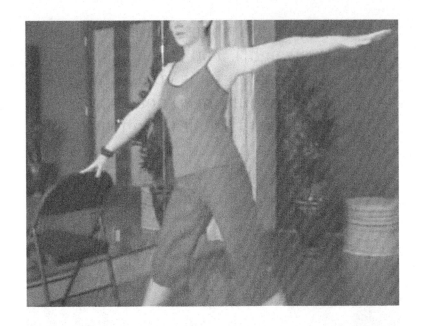

- Return to a normal standing position and repeat for ten seconds. Repeat this process on the other side.

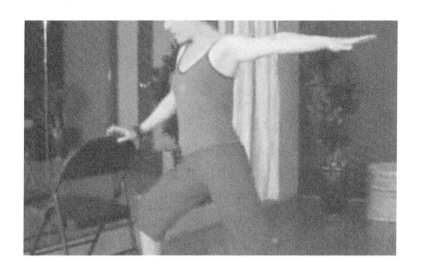

Bird Dog

To strengthen their abdominals and glutes while also improving mobility in their lower backs, this is a fantastic exercise for senior citizens. As a more advanced back exercise, the bird dog calls for a high level of balance and pre-existing strength. For added comfort and support, you can place a small pillow or blanket under your knees.

Steps:

- Put your knees up against a wall or a mattress, whichever you prefer. It is important that your knees and hips are aligned, and that your hands are directly below your shoulders

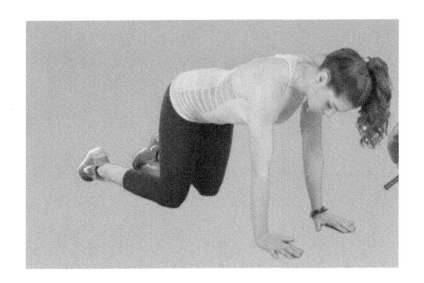

- Raise one leg behind you and extend it out straight. When lifting and straightening, do so only to the extent that you are comfortable and confident. Relax your core muscles while you inhale. Make sure your palm is level with your shoulder while simultaneously raising your other arm in front of you.

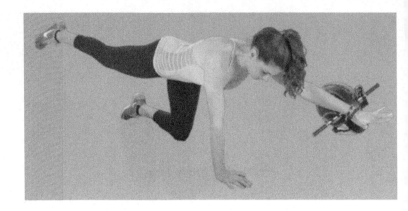

- As you return to your starting position, let go of your leg and arm and breathe out through your mouth. Move the other arm and leg in the same manner.

- To see the most progress, perform 10 repetitions of this exercise on each side, 3-4 times per week. When lifting a leg, use your abdominal muscles instead of your back muscles to avoid injuring your back.

- A more basic version of this exercise can be achieved by only lifting either one foot or one arm at the same time, rather than both legs and arms all at the same time. Bird dog is a skill you'll be able to master in due time!

Warrior 1 Yoga Pose

Warrior 1 is a more difficult challenge than Warrior 2, which was an intermediate backstretch. Both the Warrior I and II positions are excellent yoga poses for seniors to build strength and flexibility. Simply follow the steps outlined below for a proper Warrior 1 yoga asana.

Steps:

- Your toes should be facing forward as you place your feet shoulder-width apart. Keep your hands on your hips unless you need to lean against a wall, countertop, or chair for support.

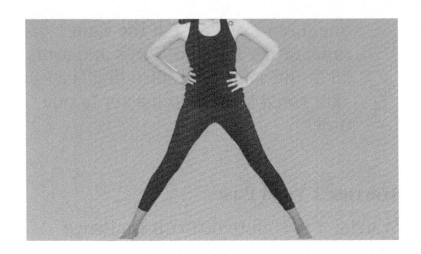

- Your right foot should be turned out straight to the right while your left foot should be turned 45 degrees to the right. Both legs must be straight for this step.

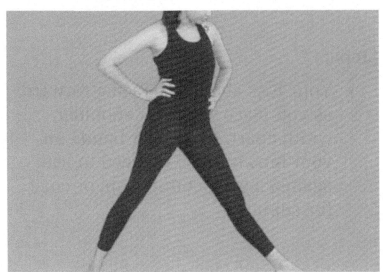

- While keeping your arms out to the sides, turn your torso and hips right. Your left foot should remain in the same position.

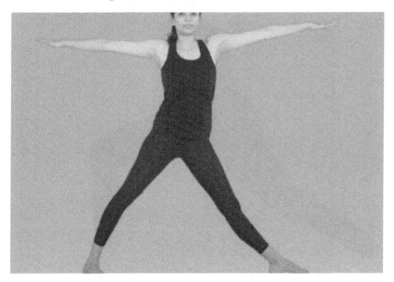

- Inhale deeply while bringing one knee up to the heart (without allowing your knee to go over the tip of your right big toe).

- When you're ready, bring your palms together and slowly bring them back down to the starting positions.

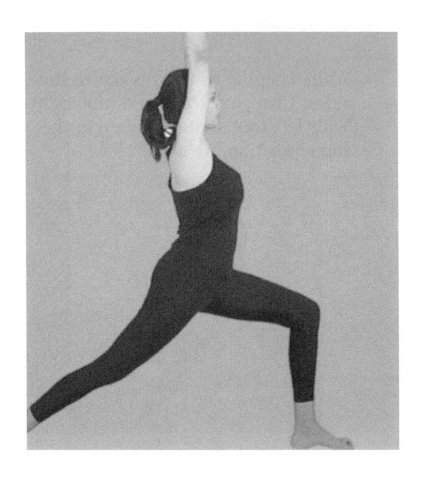

- Warrior 1 should be repeated on the other side.

Knee-to-Chest

This exercise, which appears to be simple at first glance, is quite difficult for many elderly people. If you follow the instructions carefully, you should have no trouble performing this back and hip exercise. A lot of time and effort may be required to complete this exercise, and you may also need to complete the other exercises on this list before you can do so.

Steps:

- Lie down on the floor or the bed and relax. Lie down. This exercise necessitates the use of a small pillow or blanket to support your lower back and a pillow to prop up your head.

- Keep your left foot straight and steady as you bring your right knee toward you. Grab your knee and pull it in with your hands to move closer to your chest (do not push yourself farther than you feel comfortable).

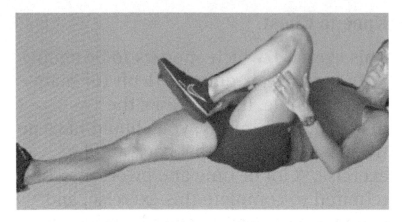

- Count to 5, then release & lightly return your leg to its initial position. In total, perform five knee-to-chest exercises on each side of your body.

Part 4

Conclusion

Preventing low back pain with regular strengthening exercises is a great idea.

Strengthening your core muscles helps you stay more stable, reduces your risk of injury, and enhances your overall performance.

Low back pain can be avoided by altering everyday activities such as squatting down to pick up items, for example.

To reap the benefits of these simple, back strengthening exercises for years to come, begin incorporating them into your daily routine today.

Made in the USA
Monee, IL
03 October 2024

67158705R00036